Heart Failure

By

Dr. Steve J. Hayes

Heart Failure

TABLE OF CONTENTS

Introduction

Heart failure treatment and safety measures. This book includes a tried-and-true, step-by-step procedure for returning a person with heart failure to an active, healthy lifestyle. Heart rehabilitation, professionally validated enzymes, and amino acids can be used to treat and prevent heart failure. This book is the first to compile the results of thousands of successful patients who recovered from heart failure successfully. Along with previously unpublished details on the essential conditions for effective heart failure rehabilitation, this book includes more than a thousand footnotes describing the clinical data he utilized to support each advice. Years of devoted research have been combined into a brief, simple guidebook. Action now is life, and knowledge is life.

Chapter 1

what causes heart failures during surgery

Myocardial localized necrosis, pneumonic embolism, electrolyte lopsided characteristics, dying, and the sedative medication given during the hour of the occasion are potential reasons for heart failure in patients having noncardiac medical procedures

Surprising heart failure during the intraoperative period adds to higher bleakness and mortality. All patients going through a medical procedure and sedation have a gamble of having a cardiorespiratory occasion perioperatively. Intraoperative heart failure is an exceptionally rare and unforeseen unfriendly occasion following a noncardiac medical procedure. Critical medical procedures, lower American Culture of Anesthesiologists (ASA) actual status, and injury are significant supporters of this undesirable occasion. 4 "H" and 4 "T" memory aides are notable reversible reasons for heart failure. A weakening in hemodynamic status during medical procedures is a mark of impending heart failure.

Patients with an okay score for the perioperative cardiovascular occasion could foster unexpected intraoperative heart failure. The groundwork for revival whenever of medical procedure is vital in the administration of abrupt and surprising cardiopulmonary capture during a medical procedure.

Intraoperative heart failure is a barely happening perilous unfriendly occasion during a medical procedure that requires prompt cardiopulmonary revival (CPR).

The event of heart failure in activity theater is diminishing in spite of a flood in the number of medical procedures each year. Each quiet who got any sort of sedation has a gamble of heart failure perioperatively yet the reason is multifactorial and complex thus, preoperative gamble separation is vital to limit this undesirable occasion. Heart failure could happen even in a patient having a lower risk score for perioperative cardiovascular occasion. At the point when a patient had intraoperative heart failure the gamble for grimness and mortality will essentially expand again placing an incredible weight on the groups of the patient and the medical services office

The huge improvements in sedation found somewhat recently added to a diminishing in perioperative difficulties including, heart unfriendly occasions.

Around the world, heart failure in non-cardiovascular medical procedures is assessed to be 13-4.3 cases per 10,000 mediations in grown-ups. Expanding in age, crisis medical procedure, comorbidities, poor useful status, and injury are as yet the best supporters of cardiopulmonary capture during sedative and careful attention. In patients who present with intraoperative heart failure, people with an ASA of III or above are liable for in excess of a lot of the cases

Myocardial dead tissue, pneumonic embolism, electrolyte awkward nature, dying, and the sedative medication given during the hour of the occasion are potential reasons for heart failure in patients having noncardiac medical procedures. The sole sedative reason for heart failure is improbable

A writing survey uncovered that intraoperative heart failure is rare in patients gone through a medical procedure utilizing provincial methods than general sedation. Patterns in the occurrence of heart failure showed an impressive decrease among patients going through a medical procedure under broad sedation, yet the recurrence of heart failure during local sedation and observed sedation was equivalent after some time

With intended for intraoperative heart failure under spinal sedation, there are a lot of case reports. A review concentrated on detail in Thailand out of 40,271 instances of spinal sedation, there were 11 heart failures, relating to a frequency of 2.73 (95% CI: 1.12-4.34) per 10,000 sedatives. There was no heart failure identified in a gynecologic patient rather 6 patients went through a cesarean segment the excess patients went through a muscular health medical procedure. Among the related elements, spinal sedation performed by a specialist is essentially connected with intraoperative heart failure however this isn't relevant in Ethiopia's arrangement, Anesthetists or anesthesiologists give a wide range of sedation to the patients

The initial 15 min of CPR is viewed as brilliant minutes for endurance since when a moment has passed mortality will be expanded by 2.1% and poor neurologic results likewise expanded by 1.2%. Around 40% will make due on the off chance that the term of revival didn't surpass 15 minutes yet simply 12% will be going to endure when over 35 minutes are taken for revival. Albeit, the length of CPR is a main consideration the hour of initiation of CPR likewise contributes extraordinarily to the result. The inability to begin CPR in the initial 2 minutes will increment mortality by 3%. Endurance will diminish by 1% - 3% at whatever point there is a 3-min defer in defibrillation or epinephrine organization after the beginning of chest pressure Taking into account the emergency unit working room as a tantamount spot for cardiopulmonary revival, a multi-focus concentrate on Ethiopia showed medical clinics are scant of fundamental hardware and medications for revival. Board for heart failure isn't accessible while all clinics remembered for the review have defibrillators. From the crisis, pharmacologic specialists, adrenaline, and atropine are accessible in all medical clinics while amiodarone, bicarbonate (sodium), and glucagon are not accessible.

Heart Failure

The inaccessibility of these medications will bring down our nature of care in the cardiopulmonary revival The board of heart failure in activity is very not the same as the external climate. Because of the plenty of reasons for heart failure, it needs a precise methodology in an organized way to in like manner act. An anesthetist and specialist should coordinate for this occasion. Accessible medications and gear should be ready in front of the patient's passage to the theater. All activity room staff should know about the circumstance and give a hand when required. Anesthetists and other staff should have satisfactory information and ability in cutting-edge life support.

Intraoperative heart failure may be a nowhere occasion. The preoperative expectation of this staggering occasion is vital however an unpredicted patient going through a generally safe medical procedure could have intraoperative heart failure. Sedation suppliers ought to continuously be ready and prepared for the administration of unexpected intraoperative heart failure. Readiness of accessible medications and gear for revival in a wide range of patients going through a medical procedure is compulsory.

Chapter 2

Heart failure after surgery

The Job of Halogenated Specialists, Myocardial Molding and Oxidative Pressure

Coronary illness requires a careful methodology here and there. Cardiovascular medical procedure patients foster cardiovascular breakdown related to ischemia initiated during extracorporeal flow. This entanglement could be diminished with sedative medications. The cardioprotective impacts of halogenated specialists depend on pre-and postconditioning (sevoflurane, desflurane, or isoflurane) contrasted with intravenous hypnotics (propofol). We attempted to put light on the shadows strolling through the line of the halogenated sedative medications' belongings in a few enzymatic courses and oxidative pressure, hanging tight for the end-product of the ACDHUVV-16 clinical preliminary with respect to the hereditary regulation of this sort of medication.

Coronary illness is a main source of mortality that regularly requires a medical procedure. In any case, patients who go through cardiovascular medicprocedure sure frequently foster cardiovascular breakdown, which is a significant reason for horribleness and mortality here cardiovascular breakdown is inclined towable ischemia incited during the extracorporeal course (EC), where a cardioplegic arrangement is implanted to cause diastolic heart failure. This confusion is related to the term EC and the standard cardiovascular status of the patient. There is a developing interest in the area of anesthesiology and postoperative basic consideration in regard to the cardioprotective impacts of myocardial preconditioning (and postconditioning) prompted by halogenated sedatives (sevoflurane, desflurane, or isoflurane) versus intravenous hypnotics (propofol)

This survey reveals a nuanced insight into the impedance systems instigated by heartbrokenness and the improvement of effector and modulator instruments prompted by using sedatives. For this reason, we investigated the job of the halogenated sedative specialists in regard to oxidative pressure, enzymatic pathways, and quality tweak (fundamentally through miRNAs).

Clinical Proof

Myocardial brokenness following cardiovascular medical procedures is a significant reason for dreariness and mortality. Ischemia initiated during the method might cause cardiovascular brokenness and low-heart yield disorder. Ischemia is initiated through actual techniques (nearby hypothermia) and the imbuement of a cardioplegic arrangement into the coronary corridors. This arrangement has a high grouping of potassium particles and diffuses inside the coronary course and cardiomyocytes, initiating heart failure and diminishing basal metabolic oxygen utilization. This arrangement can be imbued either once or a few times, in view of its creation and the kind of strategy.

Cardiovascular breakdown, when ordinary heart capability is reestablished after prompted ischemia, happens in 20% of cases. This entanglement might cause a cardiogenic shock, with high death rates [1]. At the preoperative level, cardiovascular brokenness is related to preoperative heart status, though at intraoperative and postoperative levels, heart brokenness is connected with the kind of medical procedure, the span of ischemia, and the extracorporeal course.

During the most recent 20 years, different examinations have been directed to survey the cardioprotective impacts of sedative specialists in cardiovascular medical procedures when regulated intraoperatively, postoperatively, or both.

Ischemic Pre-and Postconditioning

Specialists draw on their insight in regards to ischemic pre-and postconditioning components to actuate cardioprotection utilizing sedative specialists.

In ischemic myocardial molding, the coronary supply routes are presented to brief patterns of bracing and declamping preceding supported ischemia with the mean to decrease heart harm. Different examinations have surveyed the size of ischemic regions (areas of myocardial localized necrosis) in models presented to the method portrayed above, though, in different examinations, ischemia is prompted without past molding. The outcomes show that the size of the infarcted region was more modest in the models presented for ischemic pre-postconditioning. Ischemic preconditioning, in any case, implies a high gamble in clinical terms. Deciding the ideal term for ischemia for every patient and accomplishing cardioprotection without causing cardiovascular ischemia is testing.

Sedative Pre-and Postconditioning

To conquer the difficulties presented by ischemic myocardial molding and accomplish cardioprotection, a few creators as of late investigated the capability of sedative specialists to prompt pre-and postconditioning. This procedure mirrors ischemic molding yet forestalls the gamble of heart ischemia.

Before, during sedation acceptance, entrancing specialists were regulated with the main point of following up on the focal sensory system. As of late, in any case, attributable to their cardioprotective impacts, halogenated specialists (fundamentally, sevoflurane, desflurane, and isoflurane) have turned into the mesmerizing specialists of decision

— versus intravenous hypnotics — in the intra-and postoperative time of heart medical procedure. Early clinical preliminaries show contrasts in heart harm in light of cardiovascular catalyst levels. In clinical terms, contrasts were likewise seen comparable to the utilization of inotropic to treat the cardiovascular breakdown of low-heart yield disorder. Hence, the utilization of halogenated specialists for inhalational sedation, versus propofol, has been reported to apply cardioprotective impacts and decreased myocardial injury. In a later report, De Hert et al. archived a relationship between the span of implantation and the grouping of the halogenated specialist and its cardioprotective impacts. Conversely, late examinations question the dismalness and transient mortality results revealed for this gathering of patients corresponding to the kind of sedative regulated, yet Bonani et al. seen that unstable sedatives were better than propofol concerning long haul mortality in cardiovascular medical procedure with a cardiopulmonary detour.

As we would see it, it is extremely challenging that a solitary strategy can assist with conquering every one of the difficulties presented via heart medical procedure and further develop dreariness and mortality, no matter what the kind of method. Subsequently, the remote chance that medication might work on cardiovascular capability and diminish perioperative cardiovascular breakdown in heart medical procedures emphatically upholds its utilization.

Advancing the Clinical Utilization of Halogenated Specialists In light of the discoveries depicted over, a few examinations have been directed to decide if the supported utilization of halogenated specialists in the quick postoperative period applies comparable cardioprotective impacts as the ones seen when managed just intraoperatively, with conflicting outcomes.

Steurer et al. report a decrease in myocardial injury in heart medical procedure patients who got a halogenated specialist both intraoperatively and postoperatively (rather than propofol). The creators proposed that cardioprotection might have been accomplished through late preconditioning and postconditioning systems. Then again, Hellström et al. found no huge contrasts between treatment gatherings. It is worth focusing on that the postoperative time of sedation was very short in this review and couldn't apply the useful impacts archived in different examinations. These works evaluated early and late sedative preconditioning as well as postconditioning in heart medical procedure patients. These peculiarities are straightforwardly connected with the prompt postoperative hours.

Promising outcomes have been gotten in regards to myocardial molding actuated by halogenated specialists (sevoflurane) when regulated intraoperatively and kept up with during the quick postoperative period when contrasted with the utilization of an intravenous sedative (propofol). The supported organization of the halogenated specialist inside the initial six postoperative hours is by all accounts determinant for accomplishing cardioprotection.

Our Experience

Our examination bunch has embraced various investigations in this line of exploration. Right off the bat, we investigated contrasts among intraoperative and postoperative sedation and propofol (specialist of reference for upkeep of intravenous sedation), when contrasted with patients who got sevoflurane in the two periods. This first work uncovered that halogenated specialists applied advantageous impacts in regard to propofol. This end depended on the distinctions seen in biochemical markers of myocardial injury, heartbrokenness, and provocative reaction. This review, nonetheless, had limits corresponding to the helpful impacts of the intraoperative utilization of sevoflurane; the review didn't include a benchmark group that had just gotten sevoflurane intraoperatively and regulated another narcotic postoperatively. This implies that the valuable impacts acquired can't be straightforwardly credited to the intraoperative utilization of sevoflurane.

A subsequent report was then performed to evaluate the expected cardioprotective impacts of halogenated specialists. This study included three gatherings, one of which got sevoflurane intraoperatively and propofol postoperatively. The outcomes exhibited a decrease in the degrees of biochemical biomarkers of myocardial injury and heartbrokenness (Troponin I, NT-ProBNP), with contrasts across the three gatherings. These biomarkers were higher in the gathering that got propofol intra-and postoperatively as a sedative. Outstandingly, there were genuinely huge contrasts between the other two gatherings, proposing that cardioprotection improved when sevoflurane was directed both intra-and postoperatively.

In a later report in view of similar strategies, we investigated the potential effector components of cardioprotection applied by halogenated specialists. A clinical preliminary was led including two gatherings of patients going through a revascularization medical procedure. We tried to investigate the enzymatic instruments by which the intra-and postoperative utilization of sevoflurane applies cardioprotection. The primary gathering got sevoflurane intra-and postoperatively (SS bunch); the subsequent gathering was controlled sevoflurane intraoperatively and propofol for postoperative sedation (SP bunch); and the third gathering got propofol intra-and postoperatively (PP bunch). The outcomes uncovered that cardioprotection actuated by sevoflurane was interceded by the overexpression of the chemicals that control drug-prompted myocardial pre-and postconditioning.

The occurrence of myocardial injury (surveyed in light of plasma levels of troponin I) was lower in the gathering that got sevoflurane intra-and postoperatively. This impact is essentially connected with the height of the catalysts implied in the Gamble and SAFE (Akt/ERK 1/2/STAT5) pathways, which causes a decline in the declaration of markers of cell apoptosis (caspase3). In clinical terms, these impacts decreased cardiovascular brokenness (LCOS), which assisted protect kidneys with working.

Quality adjustment directs the outflow of a portion of the key compounds engaged with cardioprotection applied by halogenic specialists, for example, Akt, ERK 1/2, and Detail proteins, all connected with the SAFE and Hazard pathways. These discoveries urged our gathering to perform further investigations, presently on course. In these examinations, we hypothesize that sedatives would actuate myocardial molding through quality balance, subsequently directing enzymatic systems.

Non-systematizing RNA and, all the more explicitly, miRNAs, is one of the main subjects of concentrate in the field of diagnostics and therapeutics. Our gathering as of late distributed a review revealing the primer consequences of the ACDHUVV-16 preliminary. In this review, we played out the NGS sequencing of the miRNAs of cardiovascular medical procedure patients. Patients were apportioned to two gatherings in view of the intra-and postoperative sedative managed (sevoflurane versus propofol). The outcomes recognized a few miRNAs as go-betweens of cardioprotection. Be that as it may, these fundamental outcomes should be affirmed by the aftereffects of the review, which will probably be acquired by 2022.

The likelihood that sedatives prompt quality tweak with an effect on coronary illness might upset the area of anesthesiology and could include an adjustment of worldview in the enlistment of sedation and the utilization of hypnotics, which would eventually be utilized as a perioperative remedial device.

Chemical Systems of Myocardial Molding

At the cell level, reperfusion injury is portrayed by the aggregation of H+ particles, an acidic climate, calcium over-burden, and the arrangement of responsive oxygen species (ROS). These qualities bring about the launch of the mitochondrial porousness change pore (mPTP) that alters the smoothness and unbending nature of the inward mitochondrial film, impacts electron transport, and fuels mitochondrial brokenness. This prompts an endless loop that causes cell demise by delivering cytochrome C into the cytoplasm and enacting the caspase framework that instigates apoptosis. Cardiovascular molding mitigates these wounds by setting up the myocardium for ischemic affront through brief episodes of ischemia and reperfusion.

Halogenated sedatives are among the most generally utilized hypnotics because of their security profile and the consistency of their sedative impact, as well as having properties that impact heart molding. This heart molding component includes the enactment of intracellular particles and flagging pathways that at last outcome in a decline in cell oxygen interest. Various examinations have analyzed the activity components and the valuable impacts of the previously mentioned sedatives on the myocardium, managed during and after heart medical procedures, showing that mitochondria assume an essential part in them. The myocardium is a tissue rich in mitochondria that contain plenty of capabilities at the junction of cell demise or endurance, which incorporates the upkeep of vigorous ATP creation, redox flagging, calcium transport, and cell-passing pathways. Preconditioning and postconditioning triggers could share pathways for all intents and purposes for safeguarding the mitochondria, decreasing incendiary middle people, and forestalling mitochondrial calcium over-burden. A portion of the middle people of these impacts is adenosine-triphosphate-delicate potassium channels (KATP), ROS, apoptosis overflow, nitric oxide (NO), and intracellular calcium over-burden.

The mitochondrial KATP channel is a basic determinant of mitochondrial breath. Its opening incites the depolarization of the inward mitochondrial film, protecting mitochondrial volume and homeostasis. This weakens unreasonable ROS age and mitochondrial calcium aggregation that gives the ideal medium to ATP creation and restrains mPTP pore opening. This channel is an immediate objective of unstable sedatives.

Sedative Preconditioning Initiated by Unstable Sedatives Various resulting studies have tended to sedative preconditioning consequences for the myocardium utilizing enflurane, isoflurane, sevoflurane, and desflurane, planning to likewise clarify the fundamental components for such impacts. So far, proof recommends that sedative preconditioning imparts central attributes to ischemic preconditioning, giving early and postponed windows of myocardial security.

Moreover, sedative and ischemic preconditioning share a significant number of similar sub-atomic cycles engaged with myocardial security, for example, G-protein-coupled cell film receptors, intercession by means of different protein kinases, and the launch of KATP channels.

Two fundamental intracellular sign transduction pathways, guiding cardioprotection from cell-surface receptors to focalized focuses in the mitochondria, have been proposed as models to make sense of preconditioning by unstable sedatives: the reperfusion injury rescue kinases (Hazard) pathway through G-protein-coupled cell-surface receptors and the survivor-actuating factor-upgrade (SAFE) pathway.

The Gamble pathway is made out of a gathering of kinases that present cardioprotection when initiated preceding or at the hour of reperfusion. This pathway is viewed as the fundamental supportive of endurance kinase overflow and is a mix of two equal fountains: the phosphatidylinositol-4,5-bisphosphate 3-kinase (PI3K)/Akt pathway, which forestalls favorable to provocative and apoptotic occasions through the trading of signs with atomic variable kappa B (NF-kB) and glycogen synthase kinase 3β (GSK3β), and the Guide kinase 1 MEK1/ERK1/2 pathway. In short, cardioprotective announcing unpredictable sedatives are principally started by G-protein-coupled cell-film receptors, which incorporate β1-and β2-adrenergic receptors and adenosine-A1 receptors. Unstable sedatives make preparations of the sarcolemma and mitochondria KATP channels, the putative end-effectors of preconditioning, by the excitement of adenosine receptors and resulting initiation of protein kinase C (PKC) and by expanded development of NO and ROS. Actuated PKC goes about as a speaker of the preconditioning upgrade and balances out, by phosphorylation, the open condition of the mitochondrial KATP channel (the principal end-effector in sedative preconditioning) and the sarcolemma

KATP channel. The kickoff of KATP channels eventually evokes cytoprotection by diminishing cytosolic and mitochondrial Ca2+ over-burden, cell demise, and working on myocardial endurance. On account of desflurane, the feeling is finished by β-adrenergic receptors.

Enactment of PI3K brings about the phosphorylation of pyruvate dehydrogenase kinase 1 (PDK1), which initiates Akt to in this manner enlist an extensive variety of supportive endurance targets, for example, the antiapoptotic protein Bcl-2, and endothelial nitric oxide synthase (eNOS), PKC. Moreover, it phosphorylates and hinders GSK-3β, which is answerable for mPTP opening. Then again, enactment of ERK 1/2 has been proposed as an excess component by which downstream components of the PI3K-Akt outpouring might be invigorated to well regulate reperfusion injury. It has been shown that transient initiation of these Gamble kinases is defensive, setting off downstream supportive of endurance pathways, while long haul actuation is thought of as unsafe because of their development prompting impacts and enlistment of heart hypertrophy.

The significance of the Gamble pathway enacted by halogenated specialists depends on three crucial ideas: (1) the momentary initiation of its kinases is defensive; (2) actuated at the hour of early reperfusion, it produces cardioprotection; (3) it is viewed as an all-inclusive flagging fountain, a typical pathway shared by most cardioprotective treatments.

Then again, halogenated sedates likewise assume a principal part through the Protected pathway. This pathway has been depicted as an elective Gamble autonomous outpouring that intercedes cardioprotective impacts with the JAK/Detail framework. It chiefly includes cancer corruption factor-alpha (TNF-α) and the sign transducer and activator record of mitochondrial STAT3, which, while moving to the mitochondria, represses the kickoff of mPTPs and advances cardiomyocyte endurance. In people, a few distributions have underlined STAT5, for the weakening of cell passing by apoptosis, assuming an essential part in cardioprotection. SAFE potentiates its belongings through the JAK kinase, which is initially actuated by a few cytokines, including interleukin-6 (IL-6) and TNF-α. JAK will in this way actuate Detail, which will connect with NF-kB flagging that animates mitochondrial combination by the enactment of the optic decay protein (OPA1). This fountain of signs possibly influences breath and mitochondrial irritation, giving a defensive reaction. TNF-α may likewise invigorate the Protected pathway subsequent to restricting to TNF Receptor 2, which enacts STAT3. STAT3 in dimer structure has been displayed to build the counter apoptotic quality Bcl-2 and decline the apoptotic quality Bax because of a molding upgrade.

While STAT3 is a record factor, numerous STAT3 impacts in a pre-or postconditioning setting don't happen at record however are resultant of phosphorylation of different parts, for example, the phosphorylation and inactivation of the favorable to apoptotic factor Terrible. Also, it will repress the apoptotic factor forkhead box protein O1 (FOXO-1) in the core (a group of record factors that actuates the statement of apoptotic qualities). While TNF-α was initially remembered to add to reperfusion injury, it might perplexingly add to the cardioprotection instigated by pre-and postconditioning. Similarly, as with the Gamble pathway, persistent excitement of the Protected pathway is impeding the heart. In exploratory ischemic cardiovascular breakdown, the unnecessary feeling of TNF will add to the cycles of irritation, apoptosis, and heart redesigning (through TNF receptor 1). Both the Gamble and SAFE pathways have close cooperations with one another, and, in both, security in mitochondria is communicated by the hindrance of the mPTP pore and the kickoff of the KATP channel. An interrelation between the Gamble and SAFE pathways has been portrayed. For cardiomyocytes of mice lacking in STAT3 or with its inhibitor present, preconditioning systems don't secure or enact parts of the Gamble pathway like Akt and ERK. Likewise, restraint of the Gamble pathway with Akt or ERK inhibitors brings about unprotected molding techniques and the inability to actuate STAT3. Without a doubt, ERK may likewise be a vital participant in the guideline of serine phosphorylation of mitochondrial STAT3.

A few cardioprotective procedures might require initiation of the Gamble and SAFE pathways, while different methodologies might require only one of the two pathways of security.

Exploratory examinations recommend the capacity of unstable sedatives to safeguard the myocardium by sedative preconditioning altogether increments from isoflurane to sevoflurane to desflurane. The kind of unstable sedative as well as the term and recurrence of openness to the unpredictable sedative before ischemia have been demonstrated to be of expected significance in-vitro explores.

Sedative Post-Molding and Other Direct Cardioprotective Impacts Initiated by Unstable Sedatives

The second window of insurance shows up after 24 to 48 h and goes on until 72 h. It includes expanded articulation of defensive proteins, including PKCε, Detail, and NF-kB. The principal upregulated proteins engaged with postconditioning incorporate inducible nitric oxide synthase, cyclooxygenase-2, superoxide dismutase, aldose reductase, and heme oxygenase. It has additionally been proposed that the enactment of sarcolemma KATP channels, related to the mitochondrial KATP channel, lightens cytosolic calcium over-burden in the second defensive window.

Unpredictable sedatives likewise give postconditioning impacts, with efficacies like those of preconditioning as far as decreasing infarct size, when given inside the initial 30 s of reperfusion. The hidden instruments are like those of preconditioning and include the actuation of G-protein-coupled cell-layer receptors and the excitement of downstream pathways. As in preconditioning, the significant pathways implied are the Gamble and SAFE pathways.

It has been demonstrated that both Desflurane and Sevoflurane decline the outflow of Bax, a supportive of apoptotic protein, and work on the statement of Bcl-2; what's more, caspase 3 and 9 middle people of apoptosis were inactivated through the initiation of PI3K and ERK1/2. Furthermore, in mouse hearts in vivo, it has been shown that phosphorylation of the Bcl-2-related passing advertiser (Terrible) happens through the enactment of Pim-1 kinase, a proto-oncogene-intervening Akt movement in cardiomyocytes. The worldwide impact is antiapoptotic and cardioprotective, accomplishing the hindrance of mPTP opening.

Guerrero et al. have exhibited that the atomic component of the cardioprotective impact of Sevoflurane, as well as shifting a few enzymatic particles, likewise fluctuates specific miRNAs. Different key compounds in the advancement of halogenated cardioprotection are connected with their appearance through quality balance, among them, Akt, ERK 1/2, and the Detail bunch proteins, which are undeniably connected with the SAFE and Hazard pathways depicted already.

Sedative Adjustment of Oxidative Pressure in Cardiovascular Breakdown

Responsive Oxygen Species (ROS) are exceptionally receptive oxygen-containing free revolutionaries like superoxide (O_2-) and hydroxyl ($OH-$) and synthetic components, for example, hydrogen peroxide (H_2O_2) that could produce $OH-$ free extremists through the Fenton response or by consolidating with nitric oxide (NO) to frame peroxynitrite ($ONOO-$). What's more, $OH-$ could emerge from the trading of electrons somewhere in the range of O_2- and H_2O_2 through the Haber-Weiss response.

Under physiological circumstances, ROS levels are completely constrained by enzymatic or non-enzymatic cancer prevention agent safeguard frameworks. The really enzymatic safeguard frameworks are superoxide dismutase (Turf), catalase (Feline), and glutathione peroxidase (GPx). The non-enzymatic safeguard frameworks can be endogenous, characterized as those that can be blended by eukaryotic cells, or exogenous, which should be ingested with food. The most remarkable endogenous non-enzymatic frameworks are the diminished glutathione (GSH) and the Coenzyme Q10 (CoQ10), or ubiquinone, and the exogenous ones are L-ascorbic acid (Vit C), or ascorbic corrosive (AA), and Vitamin E (Vit E), notwithstanding flavonoids, beta-carotene, and lipoic corrosive.

An unevenness among ROS and cancer prevention agent guard frameworks is designated "Oxidative Pressure" and may actuate oxidative harm at the DNA level, plasmatic film, proteins, and other cellular macromolecules.

Various levels have been laid out to characterize the force of oxidative pressure. The last level has been distinguished as physiological oxidative pressure or eustress, which influences items engaged with cell digestion, and the most extreme oxidative level has been recognized as trouble, which instigates cell poisonousness through the initiation of cell cancer prevention agent safeguard processes.

Oxidative Pressure in Cardiomyocytes

In the heart, ROS contributes essentially to cell homeostasis through the guideline of cycles like cell multiplication, separation, and excitation-constriction coupling. At the point when ROS age surpasses the limit of the cancer prevention agent safeguard components or when different cell reinforcement chemicals are disabled, oxidative pressure incites cell problems at the lipid, protein, and DNA levels; harm at the sub-atomic level; and, at last, cardiovascular breakdown, myocardial redesigning with contractile brokenness, and underlying irregularities of heart tissue.

Also, in the heart, oxidative pressure might be prompted via cardiovascular hypoxia. In this present circumstance, the oxygen focus turns into a restricting variable for ordinary cell action like ATP creation, and it is related to cardiovascular harm like myocardial dead tissue, stroke, fringe blood vessel illness, renal ischemia, and ischemia-reperfusion. The myocardium, under a hypoxia condition, increments blood oxygen extraction, bringing about a significant coronary arteriovenous change, for example, the decrease in or interference of coronary blood stream, named ischemic hypoxia, or the decrease in halfway oxygen pressure (PO2) in blood vessel blood, named heart hypoxia. Oxidative pressure is perhaps the main pathway that triggers both obsessive circumstances created by their hypoxic condition of them.

Principal Wellsprings of ROS in the Heart and Their Obsessive Activity

The fundamental wellsprings of ROS distinguished in the heart are the accompanying:

The mitochondrial respiratory chain:

The primary go-betweens of ROS in mitochondria are the edifices I and III. The two buildings are answerable for the vast majority of the ROS delivered by mitochondria at the cardiovascular level, under physiological and obsessive circumstances. In examinations directed at various creature models, it has been seen that changes in the oxidative capability of mitochondria lessen heart maturing, safeguard against cardiovascular harm, and forestall left-ventricular renovating.

The compound xanthine oxide-reductase (XOR):

It is a homodimer of 30 kDa. This compound is regularly communicated in its dehydrogenase structure (XDH), yet under fiery circumstances, it changes its reductase structure to oxidase (XO). The two structures are liable for the oxidation of xanthine to uric corrosive, leaning toward a progression of electrons bound for the NAD+ decrease to NADH on account of the XDH isoform, or oxygen particles' decrease to H2O2 and O2-on account of the XO isoform. Minhas et al. have shown that the XOR protein is the primary wellspring of ROS age in the heart, and its positive guideline adds to cardiovascular hypertrophy. What's more, persistent restraint of XO forestalls oxidation of myofibrillar proteins, saving heart capability.

The protein nitric oxide synthase (NOS):

This protein has a place with a chemical bunch that catalyzes the creation of NO and citrulline from oxygen and L-arginine as substrates. Uncoupled NOS creates more ROS and less NO, changing the nitroso-redox equilibrium and causing unfriendly outcomes in the cardiovascular framework while assuming a vital part in ischemia/reperfusion injury, heart hypertrophy, and heart redesigning. On the other hand, expanded NO bioavailability might be viewed as one of the general components for cardiovascular insurance against heart weakness. In the myocardium, three NOS isoforms are communicated: endothelial NOS (eNOS or NOS3), neuronal NOS (nNOS or NOS1), and inducible NOS (iNOS or NOS2). eNOS is communicated in coronary supply routes, in endothelial cells of the endocardium, in heart drive leading tissue, and in cardiomyocytes. Myocardial nNOS is especially in the sarcoplasmic reticulum. It has been proposed that nNOS-determined NO may hinder Ca2+ deluge through L-type Ca2+ channels and animate Ca2+ re-take-up in the sarcoplasmic reticulum by advancing phospholamban (PLN) phosphorylation. The nNOS-determined NO may likewise balance the inotropic reaction to β-adrenergic excitement and repress XOR movement, in this way restricting myocardial oxidative pressure and, in a roundabout way, expanding NO accessibility inside the myocardium. At long last, NO got from the iNOS isoform is considered to negatively affect the myocardium. To be sure, upregulation of iNOS by IL-1β and IFN-γ cytokine expanded emission and has been displayed to prompt apoptosis in neonatal rodent cardiomyocytes. Also, the iNOS myocardial overexpression in mice showed cardiovascular fibrosis, cardiomyocyte demise, heart hypertrophy, and dilatation.

The NADPH-oxidase (Nicotinamide Adenine Dinucleotide Phosphate) (Nox) framework:

NADPH oxidases (Noxs) are a group of seven plasma film catalysts that address the primary wellsprings of ROS in the cardiovascular framework. They catalyze the decrease of sub-atomic oxygen to O2-involving NADPH as an electron benefactor. One of them, Nox2, is bounteously communicated in cardiomyocytes, endothelial cells, and fibroblasts. A sarcolemma compound is enacted by various improvements like angiotensin-II (Ang-II), endothelin-1 (ET-1), TNF-α, development elements, cytokines, and mechanical powers. Another compound, for example, Nox4 is constantly communicated in endothelial cells, cardiovascular myocytes, and fibroblasts and builds its demeanor in harmed heart cells.

Cytochrome P450 (CYPs) oxidase compound:

CYP isoform 2E1 (CYP2E1) is in the endoplasmic-reticulum film and is the most dynamic CYPs in ROS creation. The articulation level of CYP2E1 is essentially expanded in human-heart tissues under ischemia and is straightforwardly associated with the pathogenesis of enlarged cardiomyopathy. Its demeanor is related to an expanded articulation of oxidative pressure markers and apoptotic processes in cardiomyocytes.

The protein monoamine oxidase (MAO):

It is a protein in the outside mitochondrial film. There are two isoforms: MAO-An and MAO-B. Both isoforms take part in the guideline of digestion or debasement of catecholamines and other biogenic amines in vertebrates. Both are communicated at comparable levels in the human heart. MAO articulation and its capacity to create ROS increment with age are related to ongoing harm. Likewise, MAO-An age because of oxidative pressure triggers p53 enactment and disables lysosome capability. A hereditary erasure of MAO-B has been displayed to safeguard against oxidative pressure, apoptosis, and ventricular brokenness.

Major Cardiovascular Cell Reinforcement Frameworks Keeping harmony among oxidants and cell reinforcements shields solid life forms from the harmful impacts brought about by free extremists. The consistent age of free revolutionaries in eukaryotic organic entities should be remunerated by a comparable pace of cell reinforcement substances. Zeroing in on the heart, the three cell kinds of the myocardium (cardiovascular myocytes, fibroblasts, and endothelial cells) have the main cancer prevention agent frameworks, which are:

Superoxide dismutase (Grass):

Turf is a metalloenzyme that changes O_2-into H_2O_2 and forestalls the development of ONOO by impeding the oxidative inactivation of NO, which would cause significant obsessive results in the cardiovascular framework.

Catalase (Feline):

Feline is a tetrameric cell reinforcement protein that catalyzes the hydrolysis of H2O2 into oxygen and water. The feline is broadly circulated in the peroxisomes of the cell cytoplasm when H2O2 fixations increment, because of a provocative response.

The chemical glutathione peroxidase (GPx):

It is a cytosolic chemical that likewise catalyzes the hydrolysis of H2O2 into oxygen and water and, surprisingly, the transformation of peroxide extremists into alcohols and oxygen. Until this point, there are eight unique isoforms of GPx. The GPx-1 isoform is the most well-known. This isoform is in the cytoplasm and in the mitochondria of endothelial cells of the heart where it has been displayed to partake as a cardiovascular security component.

MiRNAs as Helpful Controllers of Oxidative Pressure in the Heart

MicroRNAs (microRNAs) are made out of 22 normally happening nucleotides that control quality articulation by matching with explicit courier RNAs, forestalling interpretation, or expanding debasement of the objective courier RNA (mRNA).

At present, miRNAs are being distinguished as a new remedial biomarker contender for various pathologies, including cardiovascular sicknesses. As referred to above, miRNAs are one of the main subjects of concentration in the field of heart impedance diagnostics and therapeutics. The primer outcomes late distributed by our gathering show a few miRNAs as go-betweens of cardioprotection in patients who got sevoflurane as a halogenated specialist in a cardiovascular medical procedure. In these patients, we have noticed varieties in the declaration of miRNAs related to better anticipation of ischemic coronary illness. These miRNAs are related to the enactment of middle people of sedative instigated pre-and post-molding, as well as cell apoptosis decrease and caspase and TNF-alpha fixations diminishing.

Ongoing distributions have portrayed the miRNAs' essential job connecting with heart illnesses, like miR-1. This miRNA is one of the most bountiful and explicit miRNAs in the heart and skeletal muscle. It is a significant controller of cardiomyocyte development in the grown-up heart, as well as a favorable to apoptotic figure myocardial ischemia, connected with sicknesses like hypertrophy, myocardial localized necrosis, and cardiovascular arrhythmias. Likewise, it tends to be utilized as a biomarker of myocardial dead tissue. Likewise, it has been shown that the statement of specific miRNAs is changed after the organization of cell reinforcement compounds, showing a defensive instrument against cardiovascular harm. Until this point in time, as per distributed examinations, miRNAs can be considered as possible targets and additional triggers of pathways connected with oxidative pressure and cardio-security.

The job of Halogenated Specialists during Cardiovascular Medical procedure

Oxygen organization is especially pertinent during and after cardiovascular medical procedures with extracorporeal courses. High oxygen focuses are regulated fully intent on forestalling cell hypoxia in patients going through a medical procedure under broad sedation and in those with intense or basic sickness. Nonetheless, the abundance of O2, or hyperoxia, is additionally known to be impeding.

At the point when ROS arrangement beats the hindrance of cancer prevention agent protection frameworks, the harmfulness produced may initiate oxidative pressure through three unique pathways: by abundance taking care of the respiratory chain and the ensuing mitochondrial uncoupling, by expanding ROS responses with NO and the subsequent age of cytotoxic receptive nitrogen species, or by lipid peroxidation, compromising the cell film strength and, thusly, its usefulness.

Then again, this produced oxidative pressure might actuate cancer prevention agent safeguard instruments through sure input meant to remunerate ROS reactivity, detoxify prooxidants, and fix the harm.

The high organization of O2 for the enlistment of sedation during surgery could produce a neurotic condition of hyperoxia. Isoflurane (2-chloro-2-(difluoromethoxy)-1,1,1-trifluoroethane) and sevoflurane (fluoromethyl-2,2,2-trifluoro-1-(trifluoromethyl) ethyl ether) are the most involved unpredictable sedatives in clinical work on giving obviousness and absence of pain. The harmfulness and gainful impacts of these medications have been broadly concentrated as well as their impact on oxidative pressure, which are all firmly connected with the visualization of medical procedures.

The relationship of the two medications with oxidative pressure and ROS creation has been dissected in different creature models of cardiovascular breakdown. As to stretch, it has been exhibited that in conditions of oxygen-focus unevenness, like hypoxia, isoflurane, and sevoflurane defensively affect ventricular myocytes, decrease the outflow of provocative variables and markers of oxidative harm, increment the statement of cancer prevention agent catalysts, for example, superoxide dismutase and catalase, direct the declaration of apoptosis-related qualities, and lessen oxidative pressure and nitric oxide levels through the ROS and NOS levels' tweak.

As to studies completed to relate the two medications to ROS creation, strangely. it has been seen that they might be engaged with the helpful impacts of unpredictable sedatives utilized in preconditioning.

Clinical examinations have likewise been directed to exhibit the cardioprotective impact of both halogenated medications, and it has been seen that they don't influence cytotoxicity nor cause they produce cell harm at the DNA level. What's more, the two sedatives are connected to the expanded movement of cell reinforcement catalyst guard frameworks and don't set off oxidative harm processes in the mediated patient or DNA oxidation. These helpful impacts of halogenated drugs work on the clinical results of patients going through heart revascularization medical procedures because of their cardioprotective impact actuated through various instruments, for example, regulation of G-protein-coupled receptors, intracellular flagging pathways, quality articulation, potassium channels, and mitochondrial capability. Likewise, the organization of unpredictable sedatives has been displayed to lessen biomarkers of myocardial harm and momentary mortality after cardiovascular revascularization medical procedures. Dharmalingam et al. as of late analyzed the connection between the unpredictable sedative organization and oxidative pressure in patients going through cardiovascular revascularization medical procedures and reasoned that preconditioning with the unstable sedatives isoflurane and sevoflurane forestalls oxidative and nitrosative pressure during heart revascularization medical procedure. Between these two halogenated specialists, isoflurane gives better insurance during the period before the cardiopulmonary detour, while sevoflurane gives assurance during the periods when the cardiopulmonary detours. As referred to above, we have exhibited that the utilization of sevoflurane during the employable and postoperative interaction builds the overexpression of compounds that decrease myocardial harm.

Then again, a few distributed examinations have scrutinized the valuable impact of unpredictable sedatives. As of late, Landoni et al. have completed a multicenter, randomized, dazed, and controlled clinical preliminary in which they saw that the utilization of unstable sedatives during cardiovascular revascularization medical procedure diminishes transient mortality in patients who went through a medical procedure; in any case, they have not noticed contrasts with respect to patients who got intravenous sedation. In this review, no review to decide the connection between the organization of both halogenated drugs and oxidative pressure was performed.

Chapter 3

Sign of a dog dying of heart failure

Congestive cardiovascular breakdown (CHF) is the point at which the heart can't siphon blood satisfactorily all through the body. This outcome in blood upholding into the lungs and liquid gathering in the body cavities, which chokes the heart and lungs and forestalls adequate oxygen stream all through the body.

In many instances of CHF, the issue isn't reversible. Here is a portion of the signs that your canine may be approaching a phase where they need hospice care or you would think about willful extermination.

What Are the Indications of a Canine Passing on from Congestive Cardiovascular Breakdown?

There are a few phases of congestive cardiovascular breakdown:

• Stage A: The canine is at high-risk for CHF, however, has no side effects and no progressions to the heart.

• Stage B1: The canine has a heart mumble yet no different signs.

• Stage B2: The canine has a heart mumble notwithstanding underlying changes to the heart, yet no clinical signs.

• Stage C: The canine has a heart mumble, underlying changes to the heart, and clinical signs related to CHF. These canines are regularly treated.
• Stage D: The canine has CHF and isn't answering standard treatments. The canine will require extraordinary treatment procedures.

The clinical finishes paperwork for CHF is comparative once a canine arrives at Stages C and D. These clinical signs that a canine is passing on from congestive cardiovascular breakdown are:

• Hacking
• Consistent gasping
• Issues breathing while inside
• Quick breathing, particularly very still
• Hesitance or refusal to work out
• Effortlessly drained subsequent to strolling and playing
• Blue-touched gums
• Enlarged mid-region
• Hacking up blood
• Breakdown

Assuming you see these indications of late-stage CHF, it doesn't mean you should quickly think about killing. A pet's side effects can determine or overseen at different stages.

For instance, hack, inconvenience breathing, and fast breathing might be treated with bronchodilators, anti-

toxins, corticosteroids, hack suppressants, ecological change (air purifiers), and even weight reduction.
Checking Your Dog's Personal satisfaction With Late-Stage CHF
As CHF advances into the hospice/palliative consideration stages (beginning at Stage C), your veterinarian will zero in on keeping up with your canine's personal satisfaction. A few inquiries that your vet might consider and examine with you include:
1. Can the canine inhale serenely all alone?
2. Does the canine appreciate feasts?
3. Does the canine appreciate cooperation with their loved ones?
4. Can the canine find time for pee and crap with nobility and rest serenely?

It's essential to check in consistently with the veterinary group to assist with keeping up with your canine's personal satisfaction. Potential complexities can come up because of sickness movement or a result of medicine. A portion of these entanglements have signs you can see, yet others will just appear in lab work at the vet's office. These may include:
• Absence of hunger
• Pneumonic edema (liquid in the lungs)
• Ascites (enlarged stomach from the liquid in the stomach pit)

• Gastrointestinal ulceration
• Uneasiness
• Loose bowels
• Weight reduction and bulk misfortune
• Changes in electrolyte blood work values:
•   Hypochloremia (low blood chloride)
•   Hyponatremia (low sodium in the blood)
•   Hypokalemia (low potassium in the blood)
•   Hyperkalemia (high potassium in the blood)
•   Kidney infection/disappointment

When Would it be a good idea for you to Euthanize a Canine with Congestive Cardiovascular breakdown?
The choice to euthanize a pet that has a congestive cardiovascular breakdown is a truly challenging and individual decision. While input from your canine's vet — , for example, blood work values, actual test discoveries, and cost — are exceedingly critical to consider, your canine's personal satisfaction and your own interests are additionally significant elements that can fluctuate enormously.

You know your pet best, and you additionally understand how you can do your pet. You likewise know when your pet is by all accounts having a truly tough time. So with regards to responding to the inquiry, "Is now the ideal time?" the reaction for your pet may be not equivalent to someone else's pet, whether or not they are encountering exactly the same thing.

Your veterinary group is there to assist you and your pet by giving help in any capacity they with canning. There is no disgrace in letting your pet go when a determination is reached. Nor is there any shame in supporting your pet until there may be every one of the more horrendous days and amazing.

Chapter 4
Strong heart failure trial

The Solid HF preliminary showed that among patients with an affirmation for intense HF, a concentrated therapy system of quick up-titration of rule coordinated medicine and close subsequent diminished the gamble of 180-day all-cause passing or HF readmission contrasted with normal consideration.

This study is meant to assess the security and adequacy of quick improvement cardiovascular breakdown treatments. 1800 patients were randomized to get either common consideration or focused energy care; with extreme focus care characterized as an increase of treatment with a beta-blocker, a renin-angiotensin framework blocker, and a mineralocorticoid receptor blocker. Security signals for cardiovascular breakdown were likewise evaluated, and biomarkers and lab measures were oftentimes estimated. Solid HF was ended right on time by the information wellbeing checking load up (DSMB) due to a fundamentally lower hazard of the essential endpoint in the extreme focus care arm when contrasted with the typical consideration arm.

The Solid HF preliminary showed that, among patients with confirmation for intense HF, an escalated therapy procedure of quick up-titration of rule coordinated medicine and close subsequent diminished the gamble of 180-day all-cause demise or HF readmission contrasted with normal consideration.

Portrayal:

The objective of the preliminary was to look at an extreme focus mediation including up-titration of cardiovascular breakdown (HF) medicines versus normal consideration among members with confirmation for intense HF.

Concentrate on Plan

The Solid HF preliminary was a global, open-name, randomized, equal gathering preliminary of members conceded with intense cardiovascular breakdown, not on full portions of HF rule coordinated clinical treatment (GDMT). Patients were randomized in a 1:1 design to extreme focus up-titration (n = 542) or common consideration (n = 536). Members were defined by left ventricular launch part (LVEF) (≤40% versus >40%). Extreme focus care required up-titration of therapies to 100 percent of suggested dosages in the span of about fourteen days of release for beta-blockers, angiotensin changing over a catalyst (ACE) inhibitors (or angiotensin receptor blockers [ARBs] assuming the patient was prejudiced to ACE inhibitors) or angiotensin receptor-neprilysin inhibitors, and mineralocorticoid receptor bad guys, and four planned short term visits over the 2 months after release with checking of clinical status, N-terminal favorable to B-type natriuretic peptide (NT-proBNP) levels, and lab values.

The review was halted early per Information and Security Checking Board's suggestion due to surprisingly incredible between-bunch contrasts.

- Complete patients screened: 1,641
- Complete randomized members: 1,078
- Concentrate on ending on September 23, 2022
- Mean patient age: 63 years
- Rate female: 39%
- Rate Dark: 21%

Consideration measures:

- Age 18-85 years
- Confirmation in no less than 72 hours prior to evaluating for intense HF
- Hemodynamically stable
- NT-proBNP >2500 pg/mL and >10% decline among screening and before randomization (yet >1500 pg/mL)
- Without treatment of ideal dosages of oral HF treatments in no less than 2 days before clinic release

Rejection measures:

- Prejudice to beta-blockers, ACE inhibitors, or ARBs

Other notable elements/attributes:

- 29% with intense coronary disorder
- 29% with diabetes

- 22% with New York Heart Affiliation (NYHA) class IV HF multi-month before clinic affirmation
- 15% with LVEF $\geq 50\%$
- Gauge LVEF: 36%
- Cardiovascular resynchronization treatment (CRT) at gauge: 1%

Head Discoveries:

The essential result, the first event of all-cause passing or HF readmission by day 180, for the focused energy care bunch versus the normal consideration bunch, was: 15.2% versus 23.3% ($p = 0.0021$).

The auxiliary result for focused energy care bunch versus normal consideration bunch:

- All-cause passing or HF readmission by day 90: 10.4% versus 13.8% ($p = 0.08$)
- All-cause demise by day 180: 8.5% versus 10.0% ($p = 0.42$)
- Change in pattern to day 90 EQ-5D visual simple scale: 0.88 versus 0.90 ($p < 0.0001$)

- HF readmission by day 180: 9.5% versus 17.1% ($p = 0.0011$)
- Changed mean change in systolic pulse by day 90: - 3.7 versus 1.6 mm Hg ($p < 0.0001$)
- Changed mean change in body weight by day 90: - 1.78 versus - 0.42 kg ($p < 0.0001$)

• Changed proportion of mathematical mean of NT-proBNP: 0.44 versus 0.56 (p = 0.0003)
Impact of EF: 68% had LVEF ≤40%. By day 90, the extent of patients randomized to extreme focus care who were up-titrated to full dosages of each of the three medication classes was 36.2% in the LVEF ≤40% bunch and 36.9% in the LVEF >40% bunch, while this extent was of 0.6% in the LVEF ≤40% bunch and of 0.0% in the LVEF >40% bunch for patients randomized to common consideration (communication p esteem = 0.97). Therapy benefit for the essential endpoint for the focused energy bunch was steady for patients regardless of benchmark EF (p for association = 0.27). Both CV demise (p for communication = 0.03) and all-cause demise (p = 0.02) at 180 days were better in the extreme focus treatment arm versus regular consideration in the gathering with LVEF >40%. These distinctions were not seen in the wake of representing Coronavirus passings. No treatment communications for HF hospitalization were noted.
The job of NT-proBNP: Patients were separated into tertiles of benchmark NT-proBNP levels into those with <2159 ng/L, 2160-4165 ng/L, and ≥4165 ng/L plasma fixations. Patients with higher NT-proBNP levels had more regrettable results yet the advantage of focused energy up-titration versus common consideration was safeguarded for the essential endpoint (p for connection by NT-proBNP tertiles = 0.20). Evaluation of the change

from predischarge to multi-week post-release of NT-proBNP fixations in the extreme focus care bunch showed a reduction ($\geq$30%) in 30%, stable qualities (between <30% decline and $\leq$10% expansion) in 43%, and an increment (>10%) in 27%. Per convention, patients with expanded NT-proBNP got more diuretics and were up-titrated all the more leisurely during the primary weeks after release. Nonetheless, by a half year, they came to 70.4% ideal GDMT dosages contrasted and 80.3% for those with NT-proBNP decline. The essential endpoint at 60 and 90 days happened in 8.3% and 11.1% of patients with expanded NT-proBNP versus 2.2% and 4.0% in those with diminished NT-proBNP (p = 0.039 and p = 0.045, separately). In any case, no distinction in result was found at 180 days (13.5% versus 11 13.2%; p = 0.93).

Translation:

The consequences of this preliminary show that, among patients with hospitalization for intense decompensated HF, quick up-titration of HF therapies in an extreme focus care model was protected and connected with a diminished gamble of death or being readmitted for HF at 180 days, regardless of standard EF or benchmark NT-proBNP. The preliminary didn't show decreases in all-cause demise at 180 days, yet this study was reasonably underpowered to distinguish such a distinction.

Enhancements in personal satisfaction, circulatory strain, and body weight were likewise noted. Serious unfriendly occasions were compared. The decreases in readmission and enhancements in personal satisfaction are of worth to the HF populace given the significant weight of illness and the dismalness related to emergency clinic stays. With the coming of more current classes of HF GDMT, there is a push for treatment with ideal dosages of GDMT. In any case, this is inadequately achieved, in actuality, clinical settings, and the proof supporting the fast commencement of GDMT was generally observational. Solid HF gives the significant, thorough preliminary proof appearance that focused energy care of members with HF to up-titrate and treat HF quickly.

Solid HF was started before the endorsement of SGLT2 inhibitors for the treatment of HF, and this drug class was for the most part not utilized in this preliminary. Nonetheless, the discoveries from this preliminary will probably likewise be appropriate to the early commencement of SGLT2 inhibitors, whose utilization has been related to optional decreases in HF hospitalization. At last, it is intriguing that the preliminary likewise incorporated a subset of members with HF with saved EF (HFpEF), where the proof for clinical treatment is substantially less hearty than for patients with HF with decreased EF (HFrEF). Extra examination assessing results by gauggaugingF will be critical to comprehend the heterogeneity of the therapy impact of the focused energy care model.

Chapter 5

Hydralazine

Hydralazine is an immediate vasodilator utilized orally to treat fundamental hypertension, among different sicknesses, and intravenously to quickly decrease circulatory strain in hypertensive criticalness or crisis. Per JNC 8 rules, it's anything but a first-line specialist for the treatment of fundamental hypertension.

For what reason is this medicine endorsed?

Hydralazine is utilized to treat hypertension. Hydralazine is in a class of meds called vasodilators. It works by loosening up the veins so that blood can stream all the more effectively through the body.

Hypertension is a typical condition and when not treated, can make harm the mind, heart, veins, kidneys, and, different pieces of the body. Harm to these organs might cause coronary illness, respiratory failure, cardiovascular breakdown, stroke, kidney disappointment, loss of vision, and different issues. As well as taking medicine, making way of life changes will likewise assist with controlling your circulatory strain. These progressions incorporate eating an eating regimen that is low in fat and salt, keeping a solid weight, practicing no less than 30 minutes most days, not smoking, and involving liquor with some restraint.

How might this medication be utilized?

Hydralazine is available as an oral tablet. It ordinarily is required two to four per day. Take hydralazine at around similar times consistently. Follow the headings on your medicine mark cautiously, and ask your PCP or drug specialist to make sense of any part you don't have the foggiest idea. Take hydralazine precisely as coordinated. Try not to take pretty much of it or take it more frequently than recommended by your primary care physician.

Hydralazine controls hypertension however doesn't fix it. Keep on taking hydralazine regardless of whether you feel good. Try not to quit taking hydralazine without conversing with your PCP.

Different purposes for this medication

Hydralazine is additionally utilized after heart valve substitution and in the treatment of cardiovascular breakdown. Converse with your primary care physician about the potential dangers of involving this drug in your condition.

This drug is at times recommended for different purposes; ask your PCP or drug specialist for more data.

What unusual precautions would it be best for me to take?

Prior to taking hydralazine,
• let your primary care physician and drug specialist know if you are susceptible to hydralazine, ibuprofen, tartrazine (a yellow color in a few handled food sources and prescriptions), some other meds, or any of the fixings in hydralazine tablets. Request your drug specialist for a rundown of the fixings.
• tell your PCP and drug specialist what other remedy and nonprescription meds, nutrients, and wholesome enhancements you are taking or plan to take. Make certain to specify any of the accompanying: indomethacin (Indocin, Tivorbex), metoprolol (Lopressor, Toprol-XL, in Dutoprol), and propranolol (Inderal LA, Innopran XL, in Inderide).
• let your PCP know if you have at any point had a cardiovascular failure, or have coronary corridor infection, rheumatic coronary illness, or heart, kidney, or liver sickness.
• Inform your primary care physician if you are expecting, want to become pregnant, or are breast-feeding. Call your primary care physician if you become pregnant while taking hydralazine.

• assuming you are having a medical procedure, including a dental medical procedure, tell the specialist or dental specialist that you are taking hydralazine.
• get some information about the protected utilization of liquor while you are taking hydralazine. Liquor can aggravate the incidental effects.

What unique dietary guidelines would it be a good idea for me to follow?

Take hydralazine with feasts or a tidbit.
Your PCP might recommend a low-salt or low-sodium diet. Follow these bearings cautiously.
How would it be a good idea for me to respond in the event that I fail to remember a portion?
Accept the missed portion when you recall it. Nonetheless, assuming that it is nearly time for the following portion, avoid the missed portion and proceed with your standard dosing plan. Avoid taking a double serving to make up for a missed one.

What incidental effects might this medicine at any point cause?

Hydralazine might cause secondary effects. If any of these adverse effects are severe or don't go away, let your PCP know:

• chest pain or discomfort that spreads to your shoulder or jaw;
• quick or beating pulses;
• a discombobulated inclination, similar to you could drop;
• agonizing or troublesome pee;
• next to zero pee; or
• sketchy skin tone.
• flushing
• migraine
• steamed stomach
• retching
• loss of craving
• the runs
• stoppage
• eye tearing
• stodgy nose
• rash

A few incidental effects can be serious. Assuming you experience any of the accompanying side effects, call your primary care physician right away:
• blacking out
• joint or muscle torment
• fever
• fast heartbeat
• chest torment
• enlarged lower legs or feet

• desensitizing or shivering in hands or feet

Would it be a good idea for me to be familiar with stockpiling and removal of this drug?
Keep this prescription in the holder it came in, firmly shut, and far away from youngsters. Store at room temperature and away from overabundance intensity and dampness (not in the restroom).
Unnecessary prescriptions ought to be discarded in extraordinary ways to guarantee that pets, kids, and others can't consume them. Be that as it may, you shouldn't wash this prescription away for good. All things being equal, the most effective way to discard your prescription is through a medication reclaim program. Converse with your drug specialist or contact your neighborhood trash/reusing division to find out about reclaim programs locally. It is critical to keep all prescriptions hidden and reach kids as numerous holders, (for example, week-by-week pill minders and those for eye drops, creams, patches, and inhalers) are not kid-safe and small kids can open them without any problem. To shield small kids from harm, consistently secure well-being covers and quickly place the prescription in a protected area - one that is up into the clouds and far away from them and reach.

If there should arise an occurrence of crisis/go too far

In the event that the casualty has fallen, had a seizure, experiences difficulty breathing, or can't be stirred, quickly call the crisis
.

What other data would it be advisable for me to be aware of?

Keep all meetings with your primary care physician and the lab. Your circulatory strain ought to be checked consistently to decide your reaction to hydralazine.

Your primary care physician might request that you check your pulse day to day. Ask your primary care physician or drug specialist to show you the ropes.

Try not to let any other person take your drug. Ask your drug specialist any inquiries you have about reordering your medicine.

You should keep a composed rundown of all of the remedy and nonprescription (over-the-counter) prescriptions you are taking, as well as any items like nutrients, minerals, or other dietary enhancements. You ought to carry this rundown with you each time you visit a specialist or on the other hand on the off chance that you are confessed to a clinic. It is additionally significant data to convey to you if there should arise an occurrence of crises.

Chapter 6

Coreg

The FDA endorses COREG, a drug of the beta-blocker family, for the treatment of mild, moderate, or severe cardiovascular breakdown.

. It assists with bringing down the pulse and making the heart siphon better. COREG can assist individuals with cardiovascular breakdown live longer and avoid the medical clinic.

What is Coreg?

Coreg is a beta-blocker. Beta-blockers affect the heart and circulation (blood flows via veins and corridors).

Coreg is utilized to treat cardiovascular breakdown and hypertension (hypertension).

Coreg is likewise utilized after a respiratory failure that has caused your heart not to siphon too.

Alerts

You shouldn't accept Coreg in the event that you have asthma, bronchitis, emphysema, extreme liver illness, or a serious heart condition, for example, heart block, "debilitated sinus disorder," or slow pulse (except if you have a pacemaker).

Try not to drink liquor somewhere around 2 hours prior to or subsequent to taking expanded discharge Coreg CR containers. Additionally try not to take medications or different items that could contain liquor. Liquor might cause the carvedilol in the controlled delivery (CR) container to be delivered excessively fast into the body. Assuming you are being treated for hypertension, continue to utilize Coreg regardless of whether you feel great. Hypertension frequently has no side effects. You might have to involve pulse drug until the end of your l

Prior to taking this medication

You shouldn't accept Coreg on the off chance that you are susceptible to carvedilol, or on the other hand assuming you have:

• asthma, bronchitis, emphysema;

• serious liver sickness; or

• a serious heart condition, for example, extreme cardiovascular breakdown, heart block, "wiped out sinus disorder," or slow pulse (except if you have a pacemaker).

To ensure Coreg is alright for you, let your PCP know if you have:

- coronary supply route infection (stopped up courses);

- slow pulses that have made you faint;

- liquid maintenance;

- asthma or other lung issues;

- angina (chest torment);

- diabetes (taking carvedilol can make it harder for you to tell when you have low glucose);

- a thyroid issue;

- kidney illness;

- dissemination issues (like Raynaud's condition); or

- pheochromocytoma (growth of the adrenal organ).

How might I take Coreg?

Take Coreg precisely as endorsed by your primary care physician. Follow all bearings on your remedy name and read all prescription aides or guidance sheets. Your PCP could occasionally alter your portion.

Coreg works best in the event that you take it with food, simultaneously and consistently.

Gulp down the drawn-out discharge case and don't pulverize, bite, break, or open it.

In the event that you can't gulp down a case, open it and sprinkle the medication into a spoonful of cold fruit purée. Swallow the combination immediately without biting. Try not to save it for some time in the future.

On the off chance that you are changed from the tablets to Coreg CR expanded discharge cases, your day-to-day complete portion of this medication might be higher or lower than previously. More established grown-ups might be bound to become lightheaded or feel faint while changing from tablets to broadened discharge cases. Adhere to your PCP's directions.

Your pulse should be checked frequently.

On the off chance that you really want a medical procedure (counting waterfall medical procedure), tell your specialist you as of now utilize this medication. You might need to take a little break.

You shouldn't quit utilizing Coreg unexpectedly. Halting unexpectedly may cause chest torment or a coronary episode. Adhere to your primary care physician's guidelines about tightening your portion.

On the off chance that you are being treated for hypertension, continue to utilize this prescription regardless of whether you feel great. Hypertension frequently has no side effects. You might have to involve a pulse drug until the end of your life.

Coreg is just essential for a total treatment program that may likewise incorporate an eating regimen, exercise, and weight control. Adhere to your primary care physician's directions intently.

Keep at room temperature and away from moisture and strong light.

What would happen if I missed a part of it?

Accept the medication in a hurry, however, skirt the missed portion in the event that it is nearly time for your next portion. Avoid taking two servings at once.

What occurs assuming that I glut?

Look for crisis clinical consideration

Go too far side effects might incorporate lopsided pulses, windedness, pale blue-hued fingernails, unsteadiness, shortcoming, swooning, and seizure (spasms).

What to stay away from

Abstain from driving or perilous action until you know what this medication will mean for you. Your responses could be debilitated. Abstain from getting up excessively quickly from a sitting or lying position, or you might feel bleary-eyed.

Coreg after effects

Get crisis clinical assistance in the event that you have indications of a hypersensitive response to Coreg: hives; trouble breathing; enlarging of your face, lips, tongue, or throat.

Call your primary care physician immediately assuming that you have:

• a woozy inclination, similar to you could drop;

• slow or lopsided pulses;

• cold inclination or deadness in your fingers or toes;

• chest torment, dry hack, wheezing, chest snugness;

• heart issues - expanding, fast weight gain, feeling winded; or

• high glucose - expanded thirst, expanded pee, dry mouth, fruity breath smell.

Normal Coreg secondary effects might include:

• tipsiness;

• slow pulses;

• the runs;

• weight gain;

• dry eyes; or

• issues wearing contact focal points.

Others may occur, as this is by no means a complete list of incidental consequences. Call your primary care physician for a clinical exhortation about secondary effects.

What different medications will influence Coreg?

In some cases utilizing specific meds simultaneously isn't protected. A few medications can influence your blood levels of different medications you take, which might increment aftereffects or make the prescriptions less powerful.

Different medications might interface with carvedilol, including solution and over-the-counter meds, nutrients, and homegrown items. Educate your PCP concerning all your ongoing meds and any medication you start or quit utilizing.

Conclusion

Heart failure is a major public health concern that has a significant impact on both the population's health and the future of healthcare. Guidelines for the management of heart failure place a strong emphasis on the progressive and gradual onset of the condition, emphasizing the critical role that upstream prevention plays in preventing heart failure episodes downstream. Prevention, Given the substantial involvement of hypertension in the anatomical and mechanical changes that result in heart failure, treatment and management of hypertension is a critical focus for preventative efforts at all stages of heart failure. It is extremely likely that we may lessen the burden of heart failure with screening, followed by early and aggressive blood pressure lowering in high-risk patients before they get clinical heart failure.